28-DAYS CH CHALLENGE FOR WEIGHT LOSS

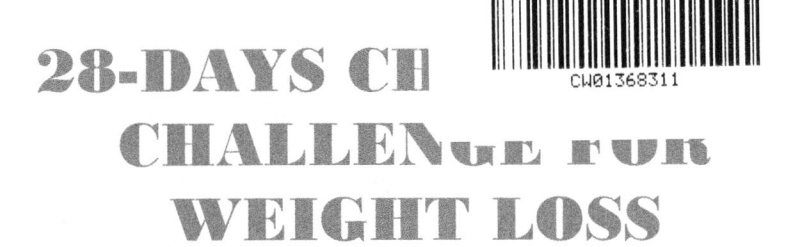

Drastically reduce your weight with this 28-days challenge!

ROGER CHEN

Copyright © 2023 Roger Chen

All rights reserved. No part of this travel guide book may be reproduced, distributed, or transmitted in any form or by any means, including photocopying, recording, or other electronic or mechanical methods, without the prior written permission of the author or publisher, except in the case of brief quotations embodied in critical reviews and certain other non-commercial uses permitted by copyright law.

Unauthorized use or reproduction of any content from this travel guide book is strictly prohibited and may result in legal action.

TABLE OF CONTENT

INTRODUCTION 5

CHAPTER 2 9

    Physical benefits of chair yoga for weight loss 9

    What to Expect from This Book 10

    How to Use This Book 10

CHAPTER 3 11

    Getting Started with Chair Yoga 11

    Overall Challenge Goals 15

CHAPTER 4 16

    Day 1: The Basics 16

    Day 2-7: Building Strength 19

CHAPTER 5 22

    Day 8-14: Improving Balance 22

CHAPTER 6 25

    Day 15-21: Burning Calories 25

CHAPTER 7 27

    Day 22-28: Mindful Eating and Portion Control 27

CHAPTER 8 32

    Maintaining Your Results 32

    Maintaining a Healthy Lifestyle Beyond the Challenge ... 33

CHAPTER 9 38

    Frequently Asked Questions about the 28 Days Challenge: Chair Yoga for Weight Loss 38

CONCLUSION 43

INTRODUCTION

In our modern-day society, where busy schedules, sedentary lifestyles, and unhealthy eating habits prevail, maintaining a healthy weight and overall well-being can be a challenging endeavor. The prevalence of weight-related health issues, such as obesity, diabetes, and cardiovascular diseases, has become a growing concern worldwide. Many people find it difficult to incorporate regular exercise into their lives due to various constraints, such as physical limitations, lack of time, or limited access to suitable fitness options.

In response to these challenges, the 28 Days Challenge: Chair Yoga for Weight Loss emerges as a practical and inclusive solution. This innovative program aims to empower individuals of all ages and abilities to embrace a healthier lifestyle through the practice of chair yoga.

Unlike traditional yoga, which often involves floor-based postures, chair yoga is a modified form of yoga that can be performed entirely while seated or using a chair for support. This makes it accessible to seniors, individuals with limited mobility, office workers, and anyone looking to embark on a fitness journey from the comfort of a chair.

Once overweight and struggling with self-esteem, Sarah stumbled upon a life-changing book titled "28 Days Chair Yoga Challenge for Weight Loss." Intrigued by the promise of a gentle yet effective exercise program, she decided to give it a try.

Each day, Sarah dedicated herself to the challenge, committing to the 10-minute chair yoga sessions. At first, it felt like a small feat, but gradually, she began to notice a shift within herself. The calming practice of chair yoga awakened a sense of mindfulness she had never experienced before.

As the days turned into weeks, Sarah's body started to transform. The gentle stretches and movements worked wonders, toning her muscles and improving flexibility. She felt her energy levels soar and stress melt away.

But Sarah's heart was moved in more ways than just the outward manifestations. The mindful eating practices taught in the book opened her eyes to a deeper connection with food. She began to savor each bite, listening to her body's hunger and fullness cues.

Slowly but surely, the pounds began to melt away, and Sarah's confidence soared. The book's meditations and relaxation exercises helped her find peace within, dispelling negative thoughts and nurturing self-love.

With newfound strength and resilience, Sarah embraced life with renewed vigor. She started exploring new hobbies, dancing and hiking with joy. Her smile became infectious, spreading positivity to those around her.

Sarah's journey with the "28 Days Chair Yoga Challenge for Weight Loss" was more than just shedding pounds—it was a transformative experience that touched her heart and soul. The book became her guiding light, leading her to discover a healthier, happier, and more authentic version of herself.

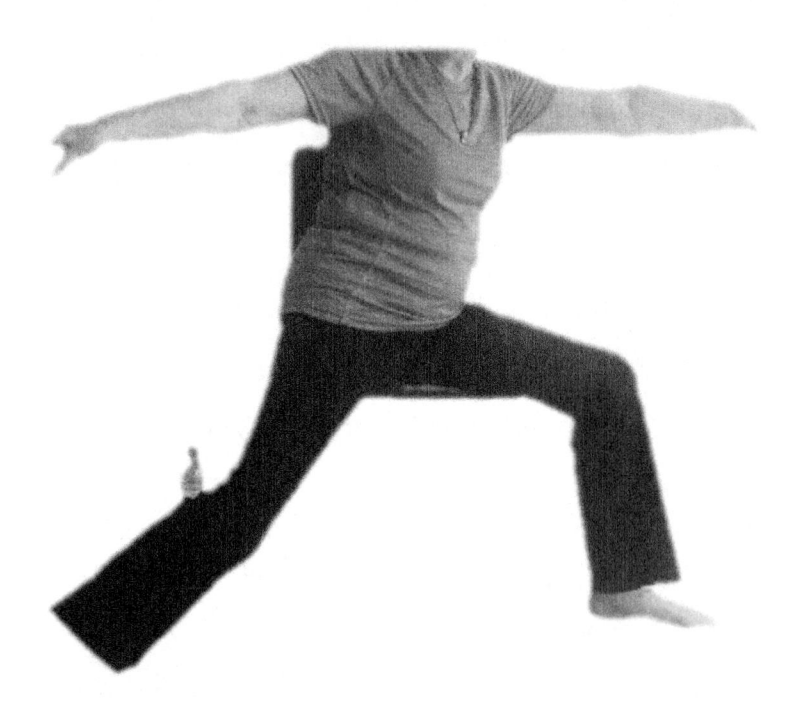

CHAPTER 2
Physical benefits of chair yoga for weight loss

1. Low-Impact Exercise: Chair yoga provides a gentle and low-impact workout that reduces the risk of injury while effectively engaging different muscle groups.

2. Increased Flexibility: Regular practice of chair yoga postures can improve flexibility, making everyday movements easier and reducing the risk of strains.

3. Enhanced Strength: Seated poses challenge muscles throughout the body, building strength and stability in the core, legs, and arms.

4. Improved Posture: Chair yoga encourages proper alignment, helping participants maintain better posture, which can alleviate back pain and reduce strain on the spine.

5. Cardiovascular Health: The dynamic movements in chair yoga can elevate the heart rate, improving cardiovascular health and aiding in weight loss.

6. Joint Health: Chair yoga can be beneficial for individuals with joint issues, as it provides gentle movement that lubricates the joints and improves mobility.

What to Expect from This Book

This book is a 28-day challenge that will help you lose weight and improve your overall health through chair yoga. Each day, you will be given a new yoga sequence to practice. The sequences are designed to be challenging but not too difficult, so you can gradually build up your strength and flexibility.

In addition to the yoga sequences, you will also find information on how to eat healthy, stay motivated, and incorporate chair yoga into your daily life.

How to Use This Book

You can use this book in a few different ways. You can follow the 28-day challenge as it is written, or you can pick and choose the yoga sequences that you want to practice. You can also use this book as a reference guide for different yoga poses and techniques.

CHAPTER 3
Getting Started with Chair Yoga

As we embark on the 28 Days Challenge: Chair Yoga for Weight Loss, it is essential to establish a strong foundation to ensure a successful and enjoyable journey. This section will guide you through the initial steps of getting started with chair yoga, providing valuable insights into the principles of chair yoga, setting goals, and creating the ideal space for your practice.

1. Understanding Chair Yoga: History and Principles

Before diving into the practice itself, it is beneficial to gain a deeper understanding of chair yoga, its origins, and the underlying principles that make it an effective form of exercise and meditation.

Chair yoga traces its roots back to the ancient practice of yoga, which originated in India over 5,000 years ago. Traditional yoga involves a series of physical postures (asanas), breath control (pranayama), and meditation to promote physical, mental, and spiritual well-being. Over time, various yoga styles and adaptations have emerged to cater to the diverse needs and capabilities of practitioners.

Chair yoga was developed as a modification of traditional yoga to make it accessible to individuals who face physical challenges, such as seniors, those with disabilities, or individuals recovering from injuries. The practice is typically performed while seated on a chair or using a chair for support, eliminating the need for complex floor-based poses. This modification allows individuals of all ages and abilities to experience the benefits of yoga, promoting overall health and wellness.

The principles of chair yoga align with those of traditional yoga, focusing on breath awareness, mindfulness, and gentle movements. The practice encourages participants to listen to their bodies, honor their limitations, and progress at their own pace. The emphasis is on creating a safe and inclusive space where everyone can experience the transformative power of yoga, regardless of their physical condition.

2. Preparing for the Challenge: Setting Goals and Expectations

As with any fitness journey, defining clear goals is crucial for success and motivation. Before commencing the 28 Days Challenge, take a moment to reflect on your reasons for embarking on this transformative experience. Are you primarily looking to lose weight, improve flexibility, manage stress, or enhance overall well-being? Identifying your goals will serve as a compass throughout the challenge, guiding your decisions and choices along the way.

Once your goals are set, it is equally important to establish realistic expectations. Chair yoga is a gentle form of exercise, and while it can yield profound results, it is essential to approach the practice with patience and an open mind. Acknowledge that progress might be gradual, and that's perfectly normal. Celebrate every milestone, no matter how small, and trust in the process of your personal growth.

3. Choosing the Right Chair and Space for Chair Yoga Practice:

A fundamental aspect of chair yoga is selecting the right chair for your practice. Ideally, the chair should have a sturdy and stable frame, with a comfortable seat and backrest. Avoid chairs with wheels, as they may be unstable during certain poses. If possible, choose a chair with a flat and level seat to ensure proper alignment during seated postures.

The space where you practice chair yoga should be tranquil and free from distractions. Choose a room with sufficient space to move your arms and legs comfortably. If possible, designate a specific area for your practice, ensuring that it is well-lit and ventilated. You may wish to add elements of calmness, such as candles, soft lighting, or soothing music, to enhance the ambiance of your practice space.

When setting up your practice space, consider having a yoga mat or non-slip surface beneath your chair to prevent it from sliding on smooth floors. Additionally, keep a water bottle nearby to stay hydrated throughout your practice.

As you prepare your space, remember that chair yoga is about creating a nurturing and non-judgmental environment. Embrace any imperfections in your practice space and allow it to become a sanctuary for self-exploration and growth.

Overall Challenge Goals

1. Weight Loss Progress: While weight loss may vary from person to person, set a realistic and achievable weight loss goal for the 28 Days Challenge. Celebrate even small increments of progress as they contribute to overall well-being.

2. Enhanced Flexibility and Range of Motion: Measure your improved flexibility and range of motion by tracking your ability to perform chair yoga poses with greater ease and comfort.

3. Reduced Stress and Enhanced Mental Clarity: Assess your stress levels and mental clarity at the beginning and end of the challenge. Notice any improvements in mood and stress management.

4. Increased Self-Awareness: Throughout the 28 Days Challenge, aim to deepen your self-awareness and connection with your body and mind. Notice how chair yoga and mindful eating practices impact your overall sense of well-being.

Remember, the 28 Days Challenge is not solely about achieving specific outcomes but also about embracing a journey of self-discovery and positive change.

CHAPTER 4
Day 1: The Basics

How to Sit Properly for Chair Yoga:

The first step to a successful chair yoga practice is to sit properly. Here are a few tips:

* Sit up straight with your back against the back of the chair.

* Keep your shoulders relaxed and your head level.

* Stand with your feet hip-width apart, flat on the ground.

* If your feet don't touch the floor, you can place a block or rolled-up towel under your feet.

Simple Breathing Exercises:

Any yoga practice should incorporate breathing exercises. They help to relax the body and mind, and they can also help to improve your overall health. Here are a few simple breathing exercises that you can try:

* **Diaphragmatic breathing:** This is the most basic breathing exercise. To do it, simply breathe in slowly and deeply through your nose, allowing your belly to expand. Breathe out slowly through your mouth, allowing your belly to contract.

* **Alternate nostril breathing:** This is a more advanced breathing exercise. To do it, place your right index finger on your right nostril and your left index finger on your left nostril. Breathe in slowly through your right nostril, then close your right nostril with your finger and breathe out slowly through your left nostril. Repeat, breathing in through your left nostril and out through your right nostril.

* **Pranayama:** Pranayama is a more advanced form of breathing that involves controlling the breath. Although there are many different pranayama practices, some of the more popular ones are as follows:

* **Ujjayi breathing:** This is a breath of fire that is used to increase energy and focus. To do it, breathe in through your nose and out through your mouth, making a slight hissing sound as you exhale.

* **Kapalbhati breathing:** This is a breath of cleansing that is used to detoxify the body. To do it, breathe in deeply through your nose and then exhale forcefully through your nose, contracting your abdomen as you exhale.

Gentle Stretches:

Once you have learned how to sit properly and you have practiced some breathing exercises, you can start to do some gentle stretches. Here are a few gentle stretches that you can try:

* **Neck stretch:** Gently tilt your head to the right, keeping your shoulders relaxed. Hold for a few seconds, then repeat on the left side.

* **Shoulder stretch:** Bring your right arm across your chest and clasp your hands together. Gently pull your right arm towards your chest, feeling the stretch in your shoulder. Hold for a short while, then do the left side.

* **Chest stretch:** Reach your arms overhead and clasp your hands together. Gently lean back, feeling the stretch in your chest. Hold for a few seconds.

* **Knee stretch:** Sit up straight and extend your right leg out in front of you. Bend your left leg and place your foot on the floor next to your right knee. Lean forward from your hips, reaching towards your toes. Hold for a few seconds, then repeat on the left side.

Day 2-7: Building Strength

On Days 2-7 of the challenge, you will start to learn some more challenging chair yoga poses that will help you to build strength. These poses include:

* **Warrior Pose:** This pose is a great way to strengthen your legs and core. To do it, sit up straight in your chair and place your feet flat on the floor, hip-width apart.

Lean forward from your hips, bringing your right arm forward and your left arm back. Maintain a straight back and a tight core. Repeat on the opposite side after holding for a short while.

* **Triangle Pose:** This pose is a great way to stretch your hamstrings and improve your balance. To do it, sit up straight in your chair and place your feet flat on the floor, hip-width apart.

Lean to the right, bringing your right arm down to the floor and your left arm up overhead. Keep your back straight and your core engaged. Hold for a few seconds, then repeat on the other side.

* **Downward Dog Pose:** This pose is a great way to stretch your back and hamstrings. To do it, start in a seated position in your chair. Place your hands on the armrests of your chair and slowly lean forward, bringing your body down towards the floor. Maintain a straight back and a tight core. Repeat on the opposite side after holding for a short while.

* **Twisted Chair Pose:** This pose is a great way to stretch your spine and improve your balance. To do it, sit up straight in your chair and place your feet flat on the floor, hip-width apart.

Twist to the right, bringing your right arm across your body and your left arm back. Maintain a straight back and a tight core. Repeat on the opposite side after holding for a short while.

* **Bow Pose:** This pose is a great way to stretch your hamstrings and improve your flexibility. To do it, start in a seated position in your chair. Place your hands on the armrests of your chair and slowly lean forward, bringing your body down towards the floor.

Grab your feet with your hands and pull your feet towards your hips. Keep your back straight and your core engaged. Hold for a few seconds, then come back up to a seated position.

These are just a few of the poses that you will learn on Days 2-7 of the challenge. As you get stronger and more flexible, you can start to challenge yourself by holding the poses for longer periods of time or by adding more challenging variations.

It is important to listen to your body and take breaks when you need them. If you feel any pain, stop the pose and try a different one.

I hope you enjoy these challenging poses and that you see some improvement in your strength and flexibility.

Here are some additional tips for Days 2-7:

* Listen to your body and take pauses as necessary.

* Start off cautiously and progressively up the intensity of your practice as you gain stronger and more flexible.

* Focus on your breathing and relax your body as you hold the poses.

* If you don't see results right away, be patient and don't give up.

CHAPTER 5
Day 8-14: Improving Balance

On Days 8-14 of the challenge, you will start to learn some poses that will help you to improve your balance. These poses include:

* **Tree Pose:** This pose is a great way to improve your balance and coordination. To do it, stand up straight in your chair and place your right foot on the inside of your left thigh.

Maintain a straight back and a tight core. Repeat on the opposite side after holding for a short while.

* **Half Moon Pose:** This pose is a great way to stretch your hamstrings and improve your balance. To do it, stand up straight in your chair and place your right foot on the floor in front of you.

Lean to the right, bringing your right arm down to the floor and your left arm up overhead. Maintain a straight back and a tight core. Repeat on the opposite side after holding for a short while.

* **Chair Pose with Arm Balance:** This pose is a great way to challenge your balance and strength. To do it, stand up straight in your chair and place your hands on the armrests of your chair. Slowly lean forward, bringing your body down towards the floor.

Bring your right arm up overhead and your left arm down to the floor. Maintain a straight back and a tight core. Repeat on the opposite side after holding for a short while.

* **Standing Forward Bend:** This pose is a great way to stretch your hamstrings and improve your flexibility. To do it, stand up straight in your chair and place your feet flat on the floor, hip-width apart.

Slowly bend forward from your hips, reaching towards your toes. Maintain a straight back and a tight core. Repeat on the opposite side after holding for a short while.

* **Warrior III Pose:** This pose is a challenging pose that requires good balance and strength. To do it, stand up straight in your chair and place your feet flat on the floor, hip-width apart.

Lean forward from your hips, bringing your right arm forward and your left arm back. Raise your right leg up behind you, keeping your knee bent. Maintain a straight back and a tight core. Repeat on the opposite side after holding for a short while.

These are just a few of the poses that you will learn on Days 8-14 of the challenge. As you get better at balancing, you can start to challenge yourself by holding the poses for longer periods of time or by adding more challenging variations.

It is important to listen to your body and take breaks when you need them. If you feel any pain, stop the pose and try a different one.

CHAPTER 6
Day 15-21: Burning Calories

On Days 15-21 of the challenge, you will start to learn some poses that will help you to burn calories. These poses include:

1. Sun Salutations: Sun salutations are a great way to warm up your body and to start burning calories. To do a sun salutation, start in a standing position with your feet together. In a pose of prayer, bring your hands together in front of your chest. Bend forward from your hips, reaching towards your toes.

Bring your hands down to the floor in front of you, then step back with your right leg into a lunge. Bring your hands back up to your chest, then step forward with your right leg to return to the standing position. Repeat on the other side.

2. Chair HIIT: Chair HIIT is a high-intensity interval training workout that is a great way to burn calories. To do a chair HIIT workout, start with a few minutes of warm-up poses.

Then, alternate between 30 seconds of vigorous chair yoga poses and 30 seconds of rest for 10-15 minutes.

3. Chair Cardio: Chair cardio is a great way to get your heart rate up and to burn calories. To do chair cardio, start with a few minutes of warm-up poses.

Then, do some vigorous chair yoga poses, such as jumping jacks, squats, and lunges. You can also do some arm exercises, such as bicep curls and shoulder presses.

4. Chair Barre: Chair barre is a great way to tone your muscles and to burn calories. To do chair barre, start with a few minutes of warm-up poses.

Then, do some chair yoga poses that focus on your legs and core. You can also do some arm exercises, such as bicep curls and shoulder presses.

5. Chair Pilates: Chair Pilates is a great way to improve your flexibility and to burn calories.

To do chair Pilates, start with a few minutes of warm-up poses. Then, do some chair yoga poses that focus on your core and flexibility.

These are just a few of the poses that you will learn on Days 15-21 of the challenge.

CHAPTER 7
Day 22-28: Mindful Eating and Portion Control

Congratulations on completing Week 3 of the 28 Days Challenge: Chair Yoga for Weight Loss! As we enter Week 4, we will shift our focus to mindful eating and portion control. This week's activities are designed to help you cultivate a more conscious and balanced approach to eating, complementing your chair yoga practice for a holistic approach to weight loss and overall well-being.

1. Cultivate Mindful Eating Habits:

Mindful eating is about paying full attention to the experience of eating and being present in the moment. It involves engaging all your senses and savoring each bite, without distractions like television, smartphones, or other electronic devices.

During meal times, take a moment to observe the appearance, aroma, and texture of your food. Chew slowly and notice the flavors as they unfold in your mouth. Pay attention to how your body responds to the food, and honor its hunger and fullness cues.

2. Recognize Hunger and Fullness Cues:

Throughout Week 4, practice tuning into your body's hunger and fullness signals. Before each meal or snack, take a moment to assess your hunger level on a scale from 1 to 10, with 1 being extremely hungry and 10 being uncomfortably full.

Eat when you feel genuinely hungry, and stop eating when you feel comfortably satisfied, around a 7 on the hunger scale. Avoid eating until you feel overly full or stuffed. By recognizing and honoring your hunger and fullness cues, you can create a more balanced and intuitive approach to eating.

3. Implement Balanced Nutrition:

Week 4 also emphasizes the importance of balanced nutrition in your diet. When planning your meals, try to incorporate a range of nutrient-dense foods, such as fresh produce, whole grains, lean proteins, and healthy fats.

Focus on colorful and vibrant foods that provide essential vitamins and minerals.

Choose whole, unprocessed foods over processed and sugary options. Eating a balanced diet will not only support your weight loss goals but also promote overall health and vitality.

To help you get started with mindful eating and portion control, here is a sample day of meals that incorporate nutrient-dense foods and mindful eating practices:

a) Breakfast:

Start your day with a nourishing breakfast. Try a bowl of oatmeal topped with fresh berries, a sprinkle of nuts or seeds, and a drizzle of honey. Savor each spoonful and notice the flavors and textures in your mouth.

b) Lunch:

For lunch, have a colorful and filling salad. Load your plate with leafy greens, cherry tomatoes, cucumber slices, shredded carrots, and avocado. Add a source of protein like grilled chicken, tofu, or chickpeas. Dress the salad with a light vinaigrette, and enjoy each bite mindfully.

c) Snack:

Choose a healthy and satisfying snack, such as a small handful of almonds or walnuts, accompanied by a piece of fruit like an apple or a banana. Take your time to chew the nuts thoroughly and appreciate the sweetness of the fruit.

d) Dinner:

Prepare a balanced dinner with lean protein, whole grains, and vegetables. For example, have baked salmon or a plant-based protein option, such as lentils or quinoa, alongside a side of roasted vegetables and a serving of whole grain pasta or brown rice. Eat slowly and enjoy the flavors and textures of your meal.

e) Dessert:

If you desire something sweet after dinner, opt for a small portion of a healthier dessert, such as a piece of dark chocolate or a fruit sorbet. Eat it mindfully, savoring the taste and indulging in the pleasure of the treat.

Throughout Week 4, aim to apply the principles of mindful eating and portion control to all your meals and snacks. Be kind to yourself, and remember that mindful eating is not about restriction but about fostering a positive and balanced relationship with food.

4. Chair Yoga for Stress Management:

Stress can significantly impact our eating habits, leading to emotional eating and overeating. To support your mindful eating journey, incorporate chair yoga practices for stress management.

During your chair yoga sessions, focus on deep, steady breathing and gentle movements that promote relaxation. Embrace poses that help release tension in the shoulders, neck, and hips, as these are common areas where stress is held.

5. Chair Yoga for Cravings and Emotional Eating:

Week 3 also addresses cravings and emotional eating. When cravings strike, halt for a moment and become aware of your feelings. Ask yourself if you are genuinely hungry or if the craving is triggered by stress, boredom, or other emotions.

Engage in chair yoga sequences that promote grounding and self-compassion. Practice seated forward bends and hip openers to release tension and connect with your emotions in a non-judgmental way.

CHAPTER 8
Maintaining Your Results

On Days 22-28 of the challenge, you will focus on maintaining your results. This will involve continuing to practice chair yoga regularly, eating healthy, and staying motivated.

Here are some tips for maintaining your results:

1. Practice chair yoga regularly: Even if you can only fit in a short practice, it is important to keep your body moving.

2. Eat healthy: Eating healthy foods will help you to maintain your weight loss and improve your overall health.

3. Stay motivated: It is important to stay motivated so that you don't give up on your health goals.

Here are some additional tips for Days 22-28:

1. If you are feeling tired or unmotivated, try a different type of chair yoga practice. There are many different styles of chair yoga, so you should be able to find one that you enjoy.

2. If you are having trouble staying motivated, find a friend or family member to join you in your chair yoga practice. Having someone to support you can make a big difference.

3. Don't be afraid to experiment with different poses and techniques. There is no right or wrong way to do chair yoga, so find what works best for you.

I hope you enjoy these final days of the challenge and that you are able to maintain your results.

Maintaining a Healthy Lifestyle Beyond the Challenge

Congratulations on completing the 28 Days Challenge: Chair Yoga for Weight Loss! As you reflect on the transformative journey you've undertaken, you may wonder how to sustain the positive changes and continue living a healthy lifestyle beyond the challenge.

This section will provide you with valuable insights and practical tips to maintain the benefits of the challenge for the long term.

1. Cultivate a Sustainable Routine:

One of the key aspects of maintaining a healthy lifestyle is creating a sustainable routine. As you move beyond the challenge, continue with your chair yoga practice, mindful eating habits, and meditation or relaxation sessions. Integrate these activities into your daily or weekly schedule, just as you did during the 28 Days Challenge.

Consistency is crucial, but remember to be flexible and compassionate with yourself. Life is full of unexpected events, and it's okay if your routine needs adjustments from time to time. The key is to find a balance that fits your lifestyle and allows you to prioritize self-care while managing other responsibilities.

2. Set Realistic and Achievable Goals:

During the challenge, you may have set specific goals related to weight loss, flexibility, or stress reduction. As you continue on your journey, consider reevaluating and refining your goals to make them realistic and achievable for the long term.

Instead of focusing solely on weight loss, consider broader health and well-being goals, such as maintaining overall fitness, improving mobility, or managing stress levels.

These goals are more sustainable and contribute to your overall quality of life beyond just a number on the scale.

3. Embrace Variety in Your Activities:

To avoid monotony and burnout, incorporate variety into your healthy lifestyle. Explore different styles of chair yoga classes or mix in other forms of physical activity that you enjoy, such as walking, swimming, or dancing. Variety not only keeps your routine interesting but also allows you to engage different muscle groups and maintain enthusiasm for exercise.

When it comes to nutrition, continue experimenting with new recipes and ingredients. Your diet should contain a variety of fruits, vegetables, whole grains, lean meats, and healthy fats. This variety ensures that you receive a wide array of nutrients to support your overall health.

4. Cultivate Mindful Eating Beyond the Challenge:

Mindful eating practices can significantly impact your eating habits and relationship with food. Continue applying the principles of mindful eating beyond the challenge by being present and attentive during meals.

Avoid distractions such as television, smartphones, or other electronic devices while eating. Instead, concentrate on how good your food tastes, feels, and makes you feel. Listen to your body's hunger and fullness cues, and eat in a way that supports your physical and emotional well-being.

5. Practice Self-Compassion and Flexibility:

The route to maintaining a healthy lifestyle will have its ups and downs. Be kind to yourself and practice self-compassion, especially during challenging times or setbacks. Remember that perfection is not the goal; progress and effort matter most.

Stay flexible in your approach to health and wellness. If your routine needs to adapt due to changing circumstances, be open to adjusting your plan while staying committed to your well-being.

6. Foster a Supportive Environment:

Surround yourself with a supportive environment that encourages your healthy lifestyle choices. Share your journey with friends, family, or colleagues who understand and respect your commitment to self-care.

Consider joining fitness or wellness communities where you can connect with like-minded individuals and gain additional motivation and inspiration. A supportive network can provide valuable encouragement and accountability as you continue your journey.

7. Regularly Reflect on Your Progress:

Set aside time for regular self-reflection to assess your progress and celebrate your achievements. Journaling can be a helpful practice to record your thoughts, feelings, and experiences on this journey.

Acknowledge the positive changes you've made and recognize the impact they've had on your well-being. Reflect on any challenges you've faced and the strategies you've employed to overcome them. Regular reflection will help you stay connected to your goals and maintain your momentum in living a healthy lifestyle

The 28 Days Challenge: Chair Yoga for Weight Loss has provided you with a strong foundation for a healthy lifestyle. As you move beyond the challenge, continue to cultivate a sustainable routine that includes chair yoga, mindful eating, and meditation or relaxation practices.

CHAPTER 9
Frequently Asked Questions about the 28 Days Challenge: Chair Yoga for Weight Loss

1. What is chair yoga, and how is it beneficial for weight loss?

Chair yoga is a gentle form of yoga that is practiced sitting on a chair or using the chair for support during standing poses. It is suitable for people of all ages and fitness levels, including those with mobility issues or limited flexibility.

Chair yoga offers numerous benefits for weight loss, including increased muscle strength, improved flexibility, and enhanced mind-body awareness. It also helps reduce stress and promote relaxation, which can positively impact eating behaviors and emotional eating patterns.

2. Do I need any prior experience in yoga to participate in the 28 Days Challenge?

No prior experience in yoga is necessary to participate in the 28 Days Challenge: Chair Yoga for Weight Loss. The challenge is designed to be accessible to beginners and individuals with limited mobility.

The chair yoga poses and sequences are gentle and easy to follow, allowing participants to progress at their own pace. The challenge also includes modifications and variations to accommodate different levels of experience and flexibility.

3. Can chair yoga help with other health conditions besides weight loss?

Yes, chair yoga can be beneficial for various health conditions beyond weight loss. It can improve overall fitness, cardiovascular health, and muscular strength.

Chair yoga is often recommended for individuals with arthritis, chronic pain, and balance issues, as it provides a safe and supportive way to engage in physical activity. Additionally, chair yoga can help reduce stress and anxiety, enhance mental clarity, and promote better sleep quality.

4. How often should I practice chair yoga during the 28 Days Challenge?

During the 28 Days Challenge, aim to practice chair yoga at least once a day, ideally for 10-15 minutes. Consistency is essential to experience the full benefits of the practice. However, if you find it challenging to practice daily, aim for at least three to four sessions per week.

The key is to make chair yoga a regular part of your routine to see progress and improvements in flexibility, strength, and overall well-being.

5. Is chair yoga suitable for pregnant individuals or individuals with specific health concerns?

Chair yoga is generally considered safe for pregnant individuals and can provide gentle exercise and relaxation during pregnancy. However, it is essential to consult with a healthcare provider before starting any new exercise routine, especially during pregnancy or if you have specific health concerns or medical conditions. Your healthcare provider can offer personalized advice and guidance based on your individual needs and circumstances.

6. How can I make chair yoga more challenging as I progress?

As you become more comfortable with the chair yoga poses and sequences, you can increase the challenge by exploring deeper variations and holding poses for a longer duration. You can also incorporate resistance bands or small weights to add resistance to certain movements, enhancing strength training. Additionally, you can explore more advanced chair yoga sequences and flows to challenge your coordination and balance.

7. Can chair yoga be a standalone practice for weight loss, or should I combine it with other forms of exercise?

Chair yoga can be an excellent standalone practice for weight loss, especially for individuals with limited mobility or those looking for a gentle and low-impact form of exercise. However, combining chair yoga with other forms of exercise, such as walking, swimming, or strength training, can further support weight loss and overall fitness goals. Variety in physical activities helps engage different muscle groups and prevents exercise plateau.

8. How can I stay motivated throughout the 28 Days Challenge and beyond?

Staying motivated during the challenge and beyond is essential for maintaining a healthy lifestyle. Set specific and achievable goals for the challenge, and regularly track your progress to stay motivated by the improvements you see. Find an accountability partner or join a supportive community to share your journey and receive encouragement. Celebrate your achievements, no matter how small, and be kind to yourself during challenging times. Remember that consistency and commitment to self-care will lead to long-term success.

9. Can chair yoga help with stress reduction and emotional well-being?

Yes, chair yoga is effective in reducing stress and promoting emotional well-being. The gentle movements, deep breathing, and relaxation practices in chair yoga activate the parasympathetic nervous system, triggering the body's relaxation response. This helps to reduce stress hormones, promote calmness, and enhance mental clarity. Regular chair yoga practice can help manage stress and improve emotional resilience.

10. How can I continue my healthy lifestyle beyond the 28 Days Challenge?

To continue your healthy lifestyle beyond the challenge, integrate the habits you've cultivated during the 28 Days Challenge into your daily routine. Maintain a regular chair yoga practice, practice mindful eating, and continue with meditation or relaxation exercises. Set new goals and keep challenging yourself to grow and improve.

CONCLUSION

The 28 Days Challenge: Chair Yoga for Weight Loss has been a transformative journey, guiding you towards a healthier and more balanced lifestyle. Throughout the challenge, you've explored the benefits of chair yoga, mindful eating, meditation, and relaxation practices. By incorporating these practices into your daily routine, you've experienced improvements in physical fitness, emotional well-being, and overall mindfulness.

Chair yoga has proven to be a gentle yet effective form of exercise, suitable for individuals of all ages and fitness levels. It has helped you build strength, flexibility, and stability while reducing stress and promoting relaxation. Mindful eating practices have enhanced your relationship with food, allowing you to make more conscious and balanced choices. Meditation and relaxation have contributed to a sense of inner calmness and self-awareness, supporting your overall well-being.

As you move beyond the challenge, it's crucial to maintain the healthy habits you've cultivated. Cultivate a sustainable routine that includes chair yoga, mindful eating, and regular meditation or relaxation sessions. Set attainable objectives with a focus on your general health and wellbeing. Embrace variety in your activities, nourishing your body with diverse and nutritious foods.

Practice self-compassion and flexibility, recognizing that the journey to a healthy lifestyle is a continuous process of growth and self-discovery. Foster a supportive environment by sharing your journey with like-minded individuals and seeking encouragement from friends, family, or online communities.

Remember that the 28 Days Challenge is just the beginning of a lifelong journey towards a healthier and happier you. Every step you take towards self-care and well-being is a step in the right direction. Embrace the joy of living a balanced and fulfilling life, knowing that you have the tools and resilience to navigate challenges and celebrate achievements.

The path to a healthy lifestyle is one of self-empowerment, self-love, and mindful choices. Take the knowledge and experiences you've gained from the 28 Days Challenge and integrate them into your daily life. Continue to nourish your mind, body, and spirit with chair yoga, mindful eating, and a compassionate approach to health and wellness.

Celebrate your progress and remember that each day is an opportunity to renew your commitment to self-care. Stay curious, stay dedicated, and stay connected to the transformational power of chair yoga and mindfulness.

CONGRATULATIONS ON COMPLETING THE 28 DAYS CHALLENGE

Printed in Great Britain
by Amazon